Beginner Guide to Everything Gluten-Free: Gluten-Free Diet and Gluten-Free Recipes

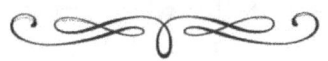

Easy Recipes, Suggestions and Guide to Eating Healthy and Cheap

By

Jamie Tyler

Introduction

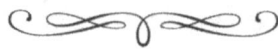

"Beginner Guide to Everything Gluten-Free: Gluten-Free Diet and Gluten-Free Recipes" is a guide for someone interested in learning basics of gluten, gluten-free diet, healthy eating, and trying easy gluten-free recipes. It is also a great introductory guide for someone suffering from **Celiac disease** who wants to understand the consequences of gluten and suggestions on eating gluten-free diet.

This book contains easy recipes, suggestions and guide to eating healthy and cheap. If you're a parent, then you'll find effective instructions, tools and recipes to start gluten-free diet in a healthy way for your entire family. If you're someone who wants to begin eating gluten-free diet, this book provides valuable introductory guidance and instructions for you.

A lot of people are talking about gluten-free diet. It seems to be the new 'fad' going around round now. 'Gluten-free' is the new label on cans and cartons. So this begs the question, do you really understand what gluten, gluten-based food products and gluten-free diets are?

What are the benefits of going for a gluten-free diet? And what exactly are the options for someone who wants to shift to gluten-free diet? That is what this book has been written for – to give you introductory information about gluten and gluten-free diets.

Thanks for downloading this book, I hope you enjoy it!

Jamie Tyler

Table of Contents

Chapter 1: What is Gluten?

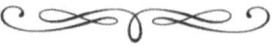

Definition:

Gluten is a form of protein that is found in some grains such as **wheat, barley, spelt and rye**. It is the substance that makes dough elastic and sticky. The word Gluten comes from Latin and means "glue".

It is also what makes foods items rise during baking, gives it shape and gives them a chewy texture. It makes dough easy to bake and prepare food. Gluten is often used in pizza, bagels, pastry products, imitation meats, beer, soy sauce, even ice cream, ketchup and pet food.

What Does Gluten Look Like?

The best example to use here would be bread or pasta. These are the best representation of what gluten looks like. Gluten is also found in most of the foods that we eat, for example pizza, spaghetti, bagels, and crackers.

It is also used to make some other food items that do not necessarily contain grains such as soup, thickeners, processed meats, meat substitutes, and instant coffee among others.

Chemically Speaking…

Chemically, it is the composite arising from two proteins – **gliadin** and **glutenin**. This composite is then attached to the starch that is stored in the **endosperm** of the cereals.

Gluten comes about during the making of dough. Glutenin molecules form minute cross-linked structures that attaches to gliadin. Gliadin in turn is responsible for the general thickness of the mix as well as its ability to stretch.

During baking, the dough is mixed with a leavening agent like yeast, which through **fermentation produces carbon dioxide gas**. This gas is in turn contained by the microscopic network, making the dough rise. When heated, the gluten coagulates and stiffens resulting in the final shape of the baked product.

Sometimes stored proteins in maize and rice are referred to as glutens. However, their proteins differ from true gluten. Generally, bread flours are high on gluten while pastry items are lower in gluten.

Who Should Avoid Gluten and Why?

According to a study, **1 in every 133** Americans suffer from **Celiac or Coliac** disease. In this condition, the immune system of an individual reacts adversely to gliadin contained in gluten. Celiac disease is **genetic**, that means that it is common with people with family history of this condition. According to a study published in 2012, an estimated **83%** of people with Celiac disease are undiagnosed or misdiagnosed.

There are also individuals who do not have Celiac disease but are sensitive to gluten. This is referred to as "**non-celiac gluten sensitivity (NCGS)**" and is also a gluten-related disorder. These individuals feel better when they're on a diet with reduced gluten. According to recent research, approximately **6%** of U.S. population may be affected by NCGS.

In addition, **Dermatitis Herpetiformis (DH)** is a skin form of Celiac disease where an individual will get extremely itchy rash triggered by eating gluten. DH can be diagnosed via biopsy of the skin.

To avoid gluten, you should be avoiding mainly following foods and drinks:

1. **Wheat**
2. **Rye**
3. **Barley**
4. **Triticale** (which is a cross between wheat and rye)

But avoiding and **limiting wheat** is challenging because wheat and its derivatives come in various names. Some wheat names that you should be avoiding are Durum flour, Spelt, Semolina, Farina, Graham flour and Kamut.

The food and drinks that are naturally free from Gluten are:

⌠ Fresh meats including fish and poultry (remember that does not include breaded, batter coated or marinated)

⌠ Fresh eggs and most dairy product

⌠ Fruits and vegetables

⌠ Seeds, beans and nuts (only unprocessed in their natural form)

In other words, being on a gluten-free diet would mean consuming meat, fish, nuts, rice, potatoes, legumes, vegetables, corn, etc. However, you need to be careful when going on a gluten-free diet as it can lack in vital **vitamins and minerals and fiber** found in wheat, barley, rye and other whole grains.

However, gluten-free diets are also a fad and have been made popular by celebrities who endorse it. A recent book by Miles Cyrus, which became New York Times Best Seller, refers to gluten as "**chronic poison**".

Chapter 2: The Effects of Gluten Based Food on Our Bodies

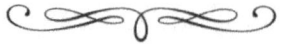

For a substance that comprises such an important dietary item, gluten has some very undesirable effects on our bodies. It is responsible for a very wide array of conditions.

First, for people with Celiac, here is a list of common signs and symptoms related to gastrointestinal conditions:

- Abdominal boating
- Abdominal pain
- Constipation
- Diarrhea
- Foul smelling & bulky stool
- Hearburn
- Irritable bowel syndrome (IBS)
- Nausea
- Vomiting
- Weight loss or weight gain

In addition, non-intestinal signs and symptoms include:

- Anemia
- Dental enamel defects, Fatigue
- Bone disease
- Depression
- Headaches
- Irritability
- Itchy skin rash
- Joint pain

- Pale mouth sores
- Infertility
- Unexplained elevation in liver enzymes

For People with Gluten Sensitivity and Celiac:

Gluten is responsible for such health conditions as bloating, diarrhea, migraine headaches, vomiting as well joint pain for a wide range of people who suffer from gluten sensitivity. **When it gets to the small intestine, immune system cell perceive the gluten as an external germ and as a result, the body begins an immune system reaction against it.** This sensitivity stimulates a stress response in the body that is markedly different from that in people who suffer from **Celiac disease**.

Celiac is a more serious condition that is characterized by the **excessive sensitivity to gluten diet**. This is an **autoimmune condition** that is inheritable and interferes with digestion in the small intestines. When the gluten gets to the small intestines for people who have Celiac, the immune system not only attacks the gluten, but also the intestinal wall tissue as well.

The intestinal wall therefore experiences damage over time and its efficiency during digestion is markedly reduced. **The person may therefore experience such symptoms as nutrient deficiency, fatigue, anemia, general lethargy as well as exposure to other diseases.** The chilling thing about Celiac is that it often has no abdominal symptoms which makes diagnosis somewhat difficult.

Diagnosis of Celiac disease:

As there are so many different types of symptoms and signs, it is difficult but possible to diagnose Celiac disease. Here are four ways this can be done:

1. **Antibody Celiac disease test:** A physician an order this test which will measure antibodies to anti-endomysium and anit-tissue transglutaminase. The antibody test will reveal patients response to gluten protein.
2. **Small intestine Biopsy:** Once the antibody tests reveal Celiac disease, patients are often advised to get a small intestine biopsy. This test will reveal whether there is damage to villi.
3. **Genetic testing:** By doing a genetic test, physicians look for HLA-DQ2 and HLA-DQ8 genes. While 95% of patients with celiac disease have DQ2 genes and 5% have DQ8, some have both.

Some Diseases Linked to Gluten Intake:

1. Dermatitis herpetiformis
2. Atopy
3. Autoimmune thyroidosis
4. Addison's disease
5. Irritable bowel
6. Inflammatory bowel disease, among others.

For People Without Gluten Sensitivity:

There is also evidence of people who neither have Celiac nor non-Celiac gluten sensitivity (NCGS) reacting adversely to gluten-based foods.

In one study, 34 people who had earlier been diagnosed with irritable bowel syndrome were chosen at random. They were put under either gluten-containing diet or diet lacking gluten. **The results indicated that the group of people who were under diet that consisted of gluten-based foods experienced worse symptoms of bowel irritation like diarrhea and bloating**.

On top of that, gluten has also been linked to several **brain disorders**. In a condition called **gluten-sensitive idiopathic neuropathy**, gluten is known to lead to or worsen many neurological illnesses.

Studies have shown that more than half of people who had unexplained mental conditions were sensitive to gluten, albeit in varying degrees. The main mental condition that is linked to gluten intake is **cerebellar ataxia** whose symptoms include difficulty with balance, motion and speech.

For most people, the mere thought of having to stop eating a gluten diet, say bread, is simply unfathomable.

Could it be that gluten is addictive? Well, you'll be surprised (or probably not) to find out that it is. Some studies indicate that gluten may posses some addictive properties. Experiments in the laboratory indicate the presence of **exorphin peptide** that has the ability to activate opioid receptors inside the brain.

The theory is that due to the increased permeability in the small intestine brought about by gluten; these exorphins may slip into the bloodstream and get to the brain. **This undoubtedly will cause addiction**.

List of food items to avoid that contain gluten:

- Wheat grain
- Barley grain or barley flour

- Rye grain or rye flour
- Oats
- Triticale grain
- Malt, malt extract, malt flavoring
- Brewer yeast
- Modified food starch made from wheat
- Dextrin made from wheat

List of packages food items that may content gluten:

- Soup
- Bouillon/broth
- Deli/lunch meat
- Salad dressings
- Soy sauce
- Teriyaki sauce
- Vegetable sauce
- Vegetable burgers
- Gravies, sauces and marinades

Non-food items that may contain gluten:

- Children's art supplies
- Personal care products (lipsticks, lip gloss etc)
- Alcoholic beverages (malt beverages, but vodka and wine are gluten-free)
- Vitamin supplements and medication

Chapter 3: What is Gluten-Free Diet and What Are The Benefits of Gluten-free Diet?

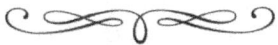

Definition:

Fortunately, there are gluten-free diets available for people who may want to avoid gluten in their diets. Gluten-free diets are basically those that do not have any foods that contain gluten. **It is the only treatment that is medically endorsed for people who suffer from Celiac disease**. This diet is also greatly beneficial for those people who suffer from other forms of gluten intolerance.

A physician will typically recommend that someone who has recently been diagnosed with celiac disease consult with a registered dietitian specializing in gluten-free diet.

A dietitian can not only assist patients with teaching them about safe gluten-free food/ingredients, identifying food that are acceptable gluten-free diets, but they can also help them find grocery stores that carry gluten-free food items.

Usually, most celiac patients on a strict gluten-free diet will experience relief from their symptoms within few weeks. But it might takes a while for the small intestines to heal.

Small number of patients still show symptoms and intestinal damage despite a strict gluten-free diet. This type of celiac disease is referred to as "**refractory celiac disease**". Researchers are currently evaluating drug treatments for this disease.

Gluten-Free Diet 101:

1. If you've just been diagnosed with celiac disease, your immediate goal is to stay gluten-free for life.
2. To begin start by easy steps, like look for dishes that require minimum customization. Perhaps just a substitution of one gluten-free item.
3. Fresh foods are great way to start gluten-free diets.
4. There are growing numbers of packages gluten-free items and meals now available in grocery stores.
5. Contact ahead when eating out to see whether the restaurant has a gluten-free selection available.
6. You will have to learn to read labels carefully.
7. As you will be limiting certain nutrient factor from your diet, remember to fill your gluten-free diet with variety of gluten-free food including fruits, vegetables, meat, poultry, fish, eggs etc.
8. A gluten-free diet may end up being high in fat and low in carbs, iron, calcium, fiber etc. Therefore people of these diets may suffer from vitamins and minerals deficiency
9. Choose gluten-free whole grain when possible like brown rice, millet, buckwheat etc
10. Ensure to eat and drink recommended amounts of milk and milk-based products. Milk provides vital source of calcium, vitamin B12 and phosphorus.
11. There is no treatment of celiac disease, simply a living a gluten-free lifestyle.

Grains and Food Items that Are Gluten-Free:

There are several grains that are considered fit for people who take gluten-free diets. Some of these are **corn, rice, millet, sorghum, beans, soya**; as well as other foods like **potatoes, fruits, vegetable and tapioca,** which is made from **cassava, yams and nuts**. In general, for a gluten-free diet, it is most important to avoid food made from wheat and barley. Therefore by avoiding wheat products (which are very common) you have already gone a long way in avoiding gluten-containing food.

Merits of Gluten-Free Diet:

There are many benefits that come with choosing gluten-free diets. Some of these benefits include **lower cholesterol levels** and **better digestive tract health**. One of the main reasons why this is so is because when people start cutting down on gluten-containing foods, they eliminate most refined foods from their diet. Foods that are refined are known to contain a lot of chemicals that are harmful to the body in the long term, their elimination from normal diet leads to improved health.

As a result, there will be a general **reduction in the intake of oily, starchy and sugary food**. One of the main sources of gluten-free diet is **fruits and vegetables**. The shift to gluten-free diet will see an increase in the consumption of these foods in place of processed and oily food. We all know that you can never go wrong with more fruits and vegetables in your diet.

For people who may suffer from Celiac disease and gluten intolerance – as well as allergy to wheat- the effects of shifting to gluten-free diet are almost immediate. The main conditions that are linked to gluten and gluten intolerance will abate or even be prevented.

Incontinence and bloating will also reduce. Patients with cases o f **Crohn's disease**, **rheumatoid arthritis** and **lupus** experience less pain and swelling of the joints. The quality of life improves markedly once the main irritant is eliminated.

Remember, if you have celiac or gluten intolerance, there is no medicine or cure for it. Take simple steps to eliminate gluten from your diet for the rest of your life. Strive to make it your lifestyle and you'll be able to conquer celiac disease and/or gluten intolerance.

Don't forget to get your free gifts when you sign up for my newsletter at the end of the book!

Chapter 4: Some Gluten-Free Diet Recipes

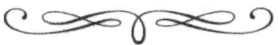

There are some recipes that you could follow when you decide to go the gluten-free way. I have divided them into breakfast, brunch, dinner as well as a few snacks for in between meals.

Breakfast and Snacks

Banana Bread
For those who just can't live without bread, here's something that you absolutely must try out.

Ingredients:

[4 cups gluten-free flour for baking
[1 ½ tsp. baking powder
[½ tsp. salt
[6 eggs
[5 big bananas, mashed
[4 tbsp. margarine
[1 ½ tsp. vanilla essence

Directions:

1. Mix the solid ingredients in one bowl; and the fluid ingredients in a different bowl. Stir in the fluid ingredients into the solid ingredients vigorously to obtain smooth batter.
2. Pour into four separate 8-in by 4-in loaf pans which had been coated with margarine afore-hand. Pre-heat the oven to 350 degrees. Put in the batter for around 50 minutes; or until a tooth pick inserted through the center comes out clean.

Spicy Crunchy Peas

This is a great Asian recipe that would serve as a nice snack between meals.

Ingredients:
- 1 cup green peas (soaked in water with baking soda)
- 5 tbsp. vegetable oil
- A mixture of salt, black salt, black pepper, coriander, pepper – all in equal proportions.

Procedure:
1. Drain all the water from the peas.
2. Put the oil on a wide pan and then add the peas when hot.
3. Initially heat at very high temp for about 12 – 14 minutes.
4. Reduce the heat then cook until crisp.
5. Remove from heat and sprinkle the mixture.

Store the remainder in an air tight container to maintain the crunchiness.

Mashed Potato Cake

Ingredients
- 200 g butter
- 200 g sugar
- 4 eggs
- 250 g mashed potatoes
- 4 lemon zest
- 1 ½ tsp. baking powder (make sure the label says gluten-free)

Directions
⌈ Mix the solid ingredients in one bowl; and the fluid ingredients in a separate bowl. Mix in the wet mixture until you obtain a mixture of smooth consistency.

⌈ Pour batter into a baking tin and put into oven pre-heated to 180 degrees Celsius. Bake for 40 minutes; or until a skewer goes through the center and comes out clean. Remove and allow it to cool.

Sorghum Porridge

This is a simple breakfast meal that takes a very short time to prepare and you are guaranteed to simply love.

Ingredients:
- 6 tbsp. sorghum flour
- 1 cup water
- 1 cup milk
- 1 tsp. margarine / butter
- Sugar or honey for sweetening (optional)

Method
- Mix the flour and a little bit of the water aside until you get a mixture of smooth and light consistency.
- Heat the rest of the water and milk until boiling.
- Pour in the mixture to the boiling water and milk while stirring consistently.
- Stir continuously until the porridge starts boiling.
- Add in the butter / margarine stir well.

Serve in bowls. Spoon some yoghurt on top and garnish with mint leaves.

There is another variation for those who love a bit of flavor.

Ingredients
- 6 tbsp. sorghum flour
- 2 ½ cups water
- 1 lemon, squeezed

Directions
⌈ Repeat as above to make a smooth mixture of water and flour of light consistency.
⌈ Heat the water until boiling.

⌈ Pour in the flour mixture while stirring continuously.
⌈ Stir until the porridge is boiling vigorously.
⌈ Pour in the lemon juice and stir well.
⌈ Sweeten with sugar or honey.

Tropical Fruit Mix
Prepare for an explosion of tropical freshness on your palate with this recipe.

Ingredients
- 1 small pineapple
- 3 bananas
- ¼ papaya
- ¼ water melon
- 1 lemon, squeezed

Directions
1. Peel the pineapple and dice.
2. Cut the banana into large chunks.
3. Peel the papaya and dice.
4. Peel the water melon and dice as well.
5. Put them all in a salad bowl and mix.
6. Drizzle in the lemon juice.
7. For best results, cover with cling film and chill before serving.

It makes great desert.

Rice bread
This is another great substitute for those who love bread.

Ingredients
- 3 cups rice flour
- 2 tsp. xanthan gum
- I tsp. gelatin (unflavored)
- 3 tbsp. sugar
- 1 tsp. salt
- 2 tsp. active yeast
- 3 eggs
- 3 tbsp. margarine

- ½ cup warm water

Directions

- Preheat the oven at 165 degrees Celsius.
- Mix the solid ingredients in one bowl, then the fluid ingredients in a separate bowl.
- Knead the dough, while making sure that the end results should vary from normal bread dough consistency to running batter. If the dough is too dry, you may add slightly warm water.
- Put the dough in a bread pan and allow it to rise until almost twice in size.
- Bake at the preset temperature until the crust gets to golden brown.
- Remove from pan and allow it to cool.

Brunch

Rice and Green Beans
This is a simple meal that you will simply love. Healthy, delicious and zero health risk. Here is for the green beans.

Ingredients
- 2 cups, green beans, boiled till well done
- 3 medium sized carrots, peeled and chopped to big chunks
- 1 medium size tomato, diced
- 1 medium size onion, chopped
- 3 tbsp. vegetable oil
- ½ tsp. cayenne pepper and salt to taste

Directions
1 Fry the oil and onion until the onions become soft and translucent.

2 Add in the diced tomatoes and stir to puree.

3 Add in the carrots, a bit of moisture (½ cup water); allow the mixture to boil and cover for a minute.

4 Next add in the beans; the seasoning and simmer for 10 minutes.

For the rice,
Ingredients
- Two cups rice
- ½ tsp. salt
- 3 1/2 cups water
- ½ cup coconut milk

Directions
a. Bring the water, coconut milk and salt mixture to a boil.

b. Add in the rice, reduce the heat and let to cook and the water to evaporate

Serve with the green beans.

Corn Bread with Vegetable and Beef

For the corn bread;

Ingredients

- 2 ½ cups of corn meal
- 1 tsp. kosher salt
- 2 tsp. baking powder
- 1 egg, beaten
- 4 tbsp. butter
- 2 cups yogurt
- 4
- 4 tbsp. sugar

Directions

a. Coat a round baking pan with butter. It should be around 8-9 inches.

b. Mix the solid ingredients in one bowl; then the fluid ingredients in a separate bowl. Mix in the liquid mixture and stir thoroughly.

c. Pour the mixture into the baking pan and bake in an oven at 400 degrees Celsius for 25 minutes or until a skewer goes through the center and comes out clean.

For the beef;

Ingredients

- 300 g diced beef
- 1 large onion, diced
- 2 large tomatoes, diced
- 1 clove garlic, crushed
- 3 tbsp. vegetable oil
- Pepper
- ½ cup water
- Salt

Directions

- Fry the onions, garlic and oil until the garlic starts sticking to the bottom of the pan.
- Add in the beef and stir until the meat surface is brown. Add in a bit of water (a few tbsp.), cover and let cook over medium low flame for 10 -15 minutes, or until the meat is well cooked.
- Add in the tomatoes and stir to puree.
- Season then add in the water. Bring to boil and simmer for 10 – 15 minutes.

Serve with the corn bread and some vegetables.

Spicy Rice with Peas Special

Ingredients
- 3 cups rice
- ½ cup green peas, priory boiled
- 4 tbsp. vegetable oil.
- Two medium size tomatoes, diced
- Three large onions, diced
- 6 medium sized carrots, diced
- 5 ½ cups water
- Salt to taste
- A mixture of the following spice, finely ground – black pepper, cumin seed. Cloves, coriander seeds

Directions
- Fry the onions until golden brown, then add in the spice mix.
- Add in the tomatoes and the peas. Stir until the tomatoes are pureed.
- Add in the carrots and the water then bring them to a boil.
- Add in the rice and enough salt to taste.
- Reduce the heat and let it boil until the rice is well cooked and the water is fully evaporated.

Serve with a sauce and vegetables as a side dish.

Dinner

Rice Noodles and Vegetables Stir Fry
This kind of noodles requires less cooking time and moisture than ordinary noodles. When overcooked, it easily becomes soggy and mushy. So care should be taken not to overcook.

Ingredients
- 250 g rice noodles
- 1 tsp. grated ginger
- 2 cloves garlic, crushed
- 1 onion, diced
- 2 baby carrots, sliced
- 1 cup, string beans
- 7 mushrooms, sliced
- Pepper and salt to season
- 4 tbsp. vegetable oil
- ½ cup lime juice
- 2 tbsp. white vinegar
- 1 chili, finely chopped

Directions
∈ Boil the noodles in salted water and remove while still slightly undercooked.
∩ Put the oil, onions, garlic and ginger into a large frying pan and start frying over medium – high heat.
∪ Add in the carrots, pepper, salt, lime juice, white vinegar and chili and let cook until the carrots are tender.
⌈. Add in the mushroom, the broccoli and pepper. Cook until the mushroom become soft and the broccoli gets bright green.
⌋. Add in the noodles and stir fry for about three minutes or until you feel satisfied with the softness of the noodles.

Serve while still hot.

Mashed Cooked Bananas and Collards

This is a nice combination for those who want to try a new flavor. First there are the mashed bananas then the collards. For the bananas;

Ingredients
- 8 raw bananas
- 2 tbsp. margarine
- ½ tsp. salt

Directions
1. Peel the bananas the boil them in slightly salted water.
2. Drain away the water. Add the salt and margarine and mash until smooth.

For the collards;

Ingredients
- 15 collard leaves, finely chopped
- 1 onion, diced
- 1 tomato, diced
- 4 tbsp. vegetable oil
- 2 tbsp. peanut butter
- A pinch of salt to taste.

Directions
  a. Fry the onion until it becomes soft and translucent.
  b. Add in the tomato and stir to puree.
  c. Add in the chopped collards and stir fry.
  d. When the collard start changing color to dark green, add in the peanut butter and salt then continue stirring for 2 more minutes.

Serve with the mashed bananas.

Spinach Special

This is a different and delicious way of making spinach that you are guaranteed to simple love.

Ingredients
- 15 spinach leaves, finely chopped
- 1 onion, diced
- 1 tomato, diced
- 4 tbsp. vegetable oil
- A pinch of salt to taste

Directions
a. Fry the onion until it becomes soft and translucent.
b. Add in the tomato and stir to puree.
c. Add in the chopped spinach and stir fry.
d. When the spinach start changing color to dark green, add in the salt then continue stirring for 2 more minutes.

Mashed Potatoes and Beef

Mashed potatoes here shall be prepared the ordinary way. I am going to give the recipe for preparing minced beef as an accompaniment.

Ingredients
- 300 g diced beef
- 1 large onion, diced
- 2 large tomatoes, diced
- 1 clove garlic, crushed
- 3 tbsp. vegetable oil
- Pepper
- ½ cup water
- Salt

Directions

⌈ Fry the onions, garlic and oil until the garlic starts sticking to the bottom of the pan.

⌈ Add in the beef and stir until the meat surface is brown. Add in a bit of water (a few tbsp.), cover and let cook over medium low flame for 10 -15 minutes, or until the meat is well cooked.

    ⌈   Add in the tomatoes and stir to puree.
    ⌈   Season then add in the water. Bring to boil and simmer for 10 – 15 minutes.

Rice and Vegetable Stew

For the rice;

Ingredients
- Two cups rice
- ½ tsp. salt
- 3 1/2 cups water
- ½ cup coconut milk.

Directions
a. Bring the water, coconut milk and salt mixture to a boil.
b. Add in the rice, reduce the heat and let to cook and the water to evaporate.

For the vegetable stew;

Ingredients
- 2 mid sized zucchini
- 2 mid size carrots
- 1 green pepper
- 1 large onion
- 2 mid size tomatoes, diced
- 2 tbsp. olive oil
- 1 cup baby corn
- 2 tbsp. cayenne pepper
- ½ tsp. salt
- 1 cup water.

Directions
a. Chop the peeled carrots, the green pepper, the onions and the zucchini into big chunks.
b. Fry the onion for a minute then add in the tomatoes. Stir to puree the tomatoes.
c. Add in the rest of the ingredients then cover for a minute to steam.
d. Add the water and the seasoning.

e. Bring to a boil and simmer for 10 minutes.
Serve with the rice.

The East African 'Matoke'
Ingredients
- 4 raw bananas, peeled
- 6 mid sized potatoes, quartered
- 1 large onions, diced
- 2 mid sized tomatoes, finely chopped
- 2 tbsp. cayenne pepper
- A pinch of salt
- ½ cup coconut milk
- 2 tbsp. vegetable oil
- 1 cup green peas, boiled.

Directions
- Fry the onions until soft and translucent.
- Add in the tomatoes and puree.
- Add in the bananas and potatoes, the coconut milk and a bit of water.
- Cover and allow it to simmer until the potatoes are almost done through.
- Add the green peas and seasoning, and then allow it to simmer for 5 minutes.

Serve while hot.

Conclusion

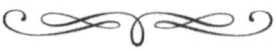

I hope this book was able to help you understand gluten and gluten-free diets. The included easy recipes, suggestions and guide were designed to make eating healthy and cheap.

I have made an effort to mainly include sources of carbohydrates and starch that do not contain gluten. This is because the main nutrient that people stand to miss out on by adopting gluten-free diet is carbohydrates.

The next step is to try out these recipes and learn about other ways to make your life much healthier.

Finally, if you enjoyed this book, then I'd like to ask you for a favor, would you be kind enough to leave a review for this book on Amazon? It'd be greatly appreciated!

Also, please sign up for my free newsletter on the next page and receive your FREE gift now!

Thank you and good luck!
Jamie Tyler

Check Out My Other Books On Amazon Kindle Store:

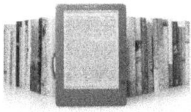

Gluten Free Meals: 50 Incredible Gluten-Free Meal Recipes for Gluten-Free Family

Gluten Free Vegan: Healthy Vegetarian Gluten Free Recipes: Vegan, Animal Free Breakfast, Lunch and Dinner Recipes

Gluten Free: Beginner Guide to Everything Gluten-Free: Gluten-Free Diet and Gluten-Free Recipes: Easy Recipes, Suggestions and Guide to Eating Healthy and Cheap

Diabetic Diet: 30-Day Lifestyle Plan To Maintain A Healthy Weight: Weight Loss And Healthy Diet Plan For Diabetics

Lose Weight: 30-Day Lifestyle Plan to Better Health by Losing Weight: What To and Not To Eat, Drink, & Making Lifestyle Changes To Look Amazing And Feel Great

Divorce With Children: Recovering From Divorce And Putting Your Life Back On Track: Dealing With Divorce, Your Ex, Children And Everything In Between

Parenting For Single Mothers: Being A Good Mom And Raising Great Kids

Raising Girls with ADHD: 20 Lessons and Tips for Parents: Tips and Strategies For Parents Dealing With Raising A Daughter With ADHD

Raising Boys With ADHD: 20 Lessons and Tips for Parents

DIY: Top 50 Hacks for Home Cleaning

Gluten Free Desserts: 50 Incredible Gluten-Free Snack Recipes for Gluten-Free Family

Sugar Free Recipes: 25 Delicious Breakfast, Lunch, and Dinner Easy Sugar-Free Recipes (Sugar Detox Diet)

Weight Watchers: Simple Quick Start Easy Recipes for Breakfast, Lunch, and Dinner

Beginner's Guide To Asperger's Syndrome: The Asperger's Syndrome Information Book (Asperger Disorder, Asperger Syndrome, Aspergers, AS, AD)

Vegan Diet For Beginners: 30-Day Vegan Diet Plan To Get You Going

Becoming A Vegan: With Everyday Guide To Plant-Based Nutrition. Includes 20 Delicious Vegan Diet Recipes

Vegan Slow Cooker For Beginners: 30 Delicious And Healthy Recipes

Lower Blood Sugar: 20 Ways For People With Diabetes To Lower Their Blood Sugar

Weight Watchers: Simple Weight Watchers Slow Cooker Recipes: 25 Healthy Weight Watchers Recipes with 7-10 Points

More Weight Watchers: Simple Weight Watchers Slow Cooker Recipes: 25 Healthy Weight Watchers Recipes with 7-10 Points

FREE Kindle Books and New Kindle Book Announcements!

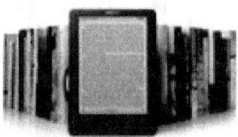

Join our exclusive readers club and receive notification when our books are FREE on Kindle Store for limited time. Also be the first to know about exciting new titles that are published every month for only $0.99.

*** We hate spam and never share your email with anyone ***

JOIN NOW!

Visit this link:
http://bit.ly/1AtBHOU

Sign Up For My Gluten-Free Lifestyle Newsletter and Receive a Free Gift!

Are you interested in receiving FREE valuable information about Gluten-free lifestyle?

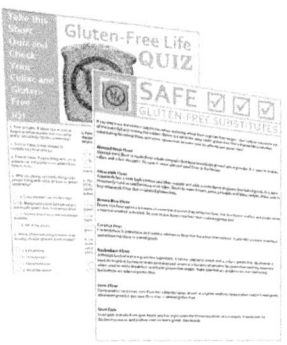

Click below to sign up for newsletter and receive these FREE gifts now!

If you sign up for my newsletter, I will be sending you gluten-free lifestyle advise, gluten-free recipes and free preview of future books about gluten-free lifestyle.

I'll even give you a gift for signing up. If you sign up now, you'll receive **FREE Gluten-Free Lifestyle Quiz.** The quiz is designed to increase your awareness and educate you about gluten-free diet and lifestyle. In addition, you'll receive a list of **Safe Gluten-Free Substitutes** that you can use in cooking and creating your own Gluten-free dishes.

Visit this link:

http://eepurl.com/2OcmP

www.ingramcontent.com/pod-product-compliance
Lightning Source LLC
Chambersburg PA
CBHW070515290526
45790CB00003B/1236